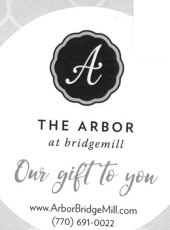

THE ARBOR
at bridgemill

Our gift to you

www.ArborBridgeMill.com
(770) 691-0022

The Journey to Senior Living

A Step-by-Step Guide for Families

Printed in the United States of America
First Printing, 2018
ISBN 978-0-692-13793-2

3715 Northside Parkway
Building 300, Suite 110
Atlanta, GA 30327
(404) 237-4026
(404) 237-1719 (Fax)

www.ArborCompany.com

CONTENTS

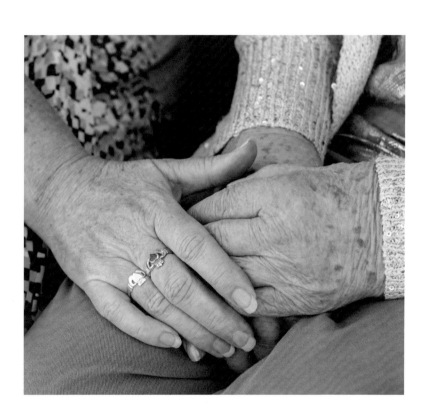

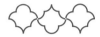

1 | *Is It Time for Senior Living?*

Whether you are already planning a loved one's move to a senior living community or just starting to consider your options, this guide has you covered.

With peace of mind, friendly neighbors, and new opportunities on the horizon, a decision to move your loved one to a community focused on senior wellness shows your dedication to their health and well-being. However, as the move draws near, you and your family may be faced with a variety of emotions. Nerves aside, if and when you decide to make a transition for your loved one, you will need to stay as prepared and organized as possible. One thing is certain: This next adventure is worth all of the packing and life changes for the older adult in your life!

WHY YOU SHOULD TRUST US

The Arbor Company operates more than 30 senior living communities across the nation, and for more than three decades, we have focused on providing quality care to seniors with a variety of abilities and challenges. Though we have won awards for some of our cutting-edge programs, we are more honored when our residents and family members say that moving into an Arbor community was one of the best decisions they ever made. Our local teams work with seniors and their families every day. We know the best parts of senior living, as well as the hard parts. We've taken families through the discussions about choosing senior care communities, and we've watched as tentative seniors become social butterflies upon move-in. We can help you through this transition.

ASSESSING YOUR LOVED ONE

Conversations about senior living are often stressful for all involved. Everyone has preconceived ideas, commitments, fears, and even associated guilt that make these conversations emotional and difficult. With such an emotionally charged topic, starting a conversation about senior living services can lead to unintended emotional issues for you and your loved ones. Before the conversation begins, take these ideas into account:

Deciding to Talk

When considering senior living, the decision is always unique to the individual. However, there are some valid shared reasons why people consider senior living. These reasons include:

- Experiencing falls at home
- Noticeable memory or judgment issues affecting daily life

- Wandering or other safety concerns regarding memory loss (leaving a hot stove unattended, becoming lost or confused, and so on)
- Lack of hygiene or personal care tasks
- Absence of nearby family or friend support system for regular check-ins
- Increased medical needs
- Increased sadness, anxiety, or worry expressed by the senior
- Inability to complete normal chores: meal preparation, medication management, light housekeeping, and so on
- Expressed or implied feelings of loneliness
- Weight loss or other nutritional concerns
- Not taking medications correctly
- Cessation of social interaction and normal routines with friends and families

Make an Honest Evaluation

As you consider the reasons why senior living might be best, take some time to evaluate your loved one's ability to handle the current situation. Does your parent need extra help that your family is unable to provide? Perhaps your loved one doesn't want to ask the family for help at all, preferring to have professional caregivers offer the assistance that he or she needs. If you are caring for a spouse with declining health, it's possible that your own health cannot handle the obligation any longer. In this case, you may feel some guilt.

Remember, though, that caregiver burnout can lead to health concerns for you, as well as other issues such as senior abuse or neglect. If you feel it's not best for your loved one to continue living at home, be honest about the reason (or reasons) why.

"Write down reasons you think that senior care may be the best option at this time."

Know Your Reasons

Before you bring up the idea of senior living, think hard about why you want to discuss it. Do you feel that the current situation is too difficult to handle? Are you worried about your own health, or do you have safety concerns (for yourself or your loved one) that make you feel anxious? Perhaps your loved one is lonely at home and wants more social interaction. Take some quiet time, a pen, and some paper to write down reasons you think that senior care may be the best option at this time.

UNDERSTANDING MEDICATION MANAGEMENT

Many seniors require the assistance of prescription or over-the-counter medications to combat symptoms of illness or pain. Even the healthiest of seniors can find themselves at the doctor's office with an infection that requires antibiotics. However, with the addition of medication to a senior's daily routine, some can take medicines incorrectly.

Seniors who make medication mistakes can face a variety of consequences, from serious to severe. Increased fall risk, increased confusion, decreased blood pressure, and even death can occur if your loved one is taking medications improperly or irregularly.

What to Look for

If you are concerned that your senior loved one could be making some medication mistakes, it is wise to watch for one or more of these red flags that could indicate mismanagement.

Inconsistent Refills

If you assist your loved one with medications—for example, picking up their refills from the pharmacy—you have the chance to notice any inconsistencies in their refill requests. Medication mismanagement can include taking too much or too little of a medicine; the frequency of your visits to the pharmacy refill counter can be an indicator that there are some issues at home.

Memory Loss or Judgment Concerns

Seniors who have a diagnosis of dementia or other memory issues are especially susceptible to medication mismanagement. If your loved ones have memory loss or judgment issues, they could be incapable of managing their own medication.

Medications that Look the Same

One of the biggest contributors to medication mistakes in the senior population is the confusion of one medication for another. Similar-looking medications can exacerbate this problem for even the most detail-oriented senior. If two or more of your loved one's medications look similar to you, this could be an indicator that a potential mistake is on the horizon.

Too Many Supplements or Over-the-Counter Medications

Drug interactions can happen quickly and without warning, especially if a prescribing doctor does not know which supplements or over-the-counter medications are also being taken. If your loved one has a medicine cabinet overflowing with vitamins or over-the-counter medications, beware. Make an appointment to talk with your loved one's doctor, as well as the care staff at the assisted living community where he or she resides, about any nonprescription medications taken on a daily basis.

Fine Motor Concerns

Seniors with decreasing fine motor skills can find opening pill packets or bottles nearly impossible. If your loved one becomes frustrated or has difficulty getting ready to take their medications, it could result in a problem of skipping doses.

What to Do Next

Managing medications at home is difficult for most seniors, especially if there are multiple prescriptions to monitor. Without direct oversight from a caring family member or a professional, mistakes happen frequently and can be devastating. Fortunately, many senior living communities offer peace of mind through their medication management programs.

In senior living communities, residents receive medications from a trained professional. This not only eliminates stress and frustration for the senior, but also keeps the senior safer and healthier than if they managed their medications alone at home.

*"Take some time to step back and gather
reliable facts; these can reassure you in your
preparations to initiate the talk confidently."*

If you are concerned about medication management for your
loved one, or if you noticed one or more red flags during your
last visit, it is time to chat with your loved one about your
concerns. Make an appointment with your loved one's doctor as
well to openly discuss senior living community options. Living in
such a community could literally save your loved one's life.

HAVING THE CONVERSATION

If you have noticed some decline in the health of your spouse
or senior parent, it can be tempting to quickly jump into a
conversation. However, some forethought is required before you
bring up the subject. Take some time to step back and gather
reliable facts; these can reassure you in your preparations to
initiate the talk confidently.

Get the Facts About Senior Living

Before you start, it's important to gather all the facts about your
options. Senior living communities come in all shapes and sizes,
serving seniors of many different abilities and interests. Perhaps
you already know that senior living is appealing, but anticipate

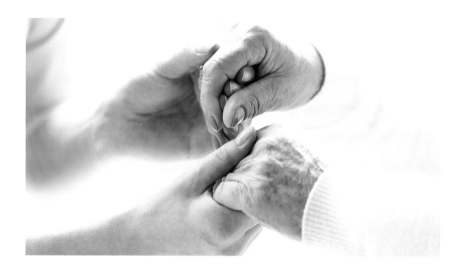

pushback from other family members, especially because they may have biases against their perception of "nursing homes."

Many people have misconceptions about senior living. These can come from past experiences, old memories, or even stereotypes portrayed in television and movies. Before attempting to convince your family, arm yourself with facts about the senior living option or options that you have in mind, whether it be independent living, assisted living, memory care, or skilled nursing.

Senior living communities have undergone major culture changes over the past few decades, cementing the fact that these communities are no longer stereotypical nursing homes. These are just a few items to keep in mind when considering senior living:

- **It's not just bingo!** Senior living communities feature daily activities and events for residents, ranging from travel opportunities and yoga to community college lectures and Elvis impersonator socials.

- **There is choice!** Communities focus on giving residents options for their environment, from the arrival time of housekeeping services during the week to entrée choices at mealtimes.

- **Socialization keeps residents healthier and happier!** Isolation is a major factor when it comes to the emotional, physical, and cognitive health issues in seniors who live at home without regular socialization. With neighbors and staff members just steps away at a senior living community, residents are more likely to stay active, engaged, and ultimately healthier.

- **Connection is encouraged!** Residents are encouraged to connect with their peers and greater community as much as they are able—through social media, group activities, volunteer activities, and planned trips.

After you have taken some time to step back and evaluate the reasons why you believe senior living is a good option to discuss, organize your thoughts so that you are ready to express your point of view before the talk even begins. Going into the process prepared, both emotionally and intellectually, can help you keep your tone appropriate and levelheaded.

Prepare with Clarity

Although it's not alway realistic to make a word-for-word script before the meeting, writing out a few key talking points can help you articulate your feelings and worries appropriately. Remember to consider your audience as well; phrase your feelings and thoughts in such a way that they will be understood and well-received.

Consider Others' Feelings

If you are preparing to talk with your loved one about why you think they need some extra assistance, keep their feelings in mind and at the forefront of your agenda. The conversation can feel embarrassing, humbling, and even scary for your loved one. If you are ready to tell your children that you want to move to a senior community, you may be met with feelings of worry or guilt on their part. Make their feelings a priority when considering what you will say, and phrase your feelings in a way that can give them the greatest chance of being heard. Keep your tone honest, objective, and caring.

Prepare with an Outline

Prepare an outline or checklist to keep yourself on task during your talk. If the situation becomes emotional, or if you find yourself veering off topic, you can easily look down at your outline to get back on track and ensure that you are covering what you feel like you need to say during your conversation. That said, don't make the outline or list of items to cover too long; instead, pick a few items and use those as examples to illustrate your point.

Discuss and Plan with Other Family Members or Caregivers

You may find yourself in a position of not only having to convince your loved one that senior care is the best option, but also having to convince children or other invested family members that the decision is sound. In this case, you must walk a fine line of expressing your own concerns while balancing the feelings and opinions of others in the room. Consider making a plan for the discussion ahead of time, and bring with you any necessary support to keep yourself levelheaded and heard.

"Bring with you any necessary support to keep yourself levelheaded and heard."

Time for the Talk

Ensure that you are as prepared and informed as possible and that you are ready to broach the subject of senior living to your loved one and other family members.

Introduce the Topic of Senior Living

Introducing the topic of senior living in a positive way and at a good time can be half the battle. Be conscious of the timing of your discussion. Avoid bringing up your concerns during a high-stress moment or when the time doesn't allow for good discussion. For example, Thanksgiving dinner with the whole family may not be the best time to address your spouse's memory loss. Plan ahead for a time when interested parties can come together for a serious talk.

Be Prepared for Strong Emotions

You may have been considering senior living for a while, but your loved one and other family members likely haven't been, so your decision may seem abrupt. Even if you phrase it kindly, emotions can get the best of everyone and lead to unintended feelings of guilt or worry. Don't let negative reactions keep you from gently continuing your conversation, but be sure that you are taking ample time to listen to everyone's feelings.

Don't Be Pushy

If you are met with negative responses or a loved one who immediately goes on the defensive, resist the urge to continue pushing your views or concerns in the same way. Just because you have taken time to research and reflect on the best options for the future doesn't mean that everyone will instantly agree with you. Adapt your approach to fit the mood of the room, while remaining gentle, kind, and persistent. Allow everyone to be part of the decision.

If you are having this conversation with a group of people, the dynamics of the room can vary greatly. If there are others present who share your viewpoint, it can be easy to work together and tear down those that disagree with your ideas. This is especially common in family relationships as everyone reverts into their traditional family roles. Resist the urge to gang up on those who do not share your opinions, instead opting for a gracious and attentive attitude.

Talk Through Why the Decision Is Best for Your Loved One

Listening to the opinions and thoughts of others in the room is imperative, but this does not mean that your opinion needs to change. If you are sure this is the best decision, be firm in your stance for senior living assistance. However, understand that you may not be able to sway everyone in the room to your position with one conversation, no matter how well executed. It may take many conversations—and even the assistance of a professional, such as a geriatrician or trusted doctor—before everyone gets on board with this tough decision.

AFTER THE TALK

With the initial talk finally over, you are most likely not yet done with the conversation. Multiple conversations might be necessary before your family can reach an amicable and responsible decision. For better or for worse, you are a family, and a family puts the needs of aging loved ones at the center of difficult conversations and decisions. You are not the first family to have these conversations, and you will not be the last. Choose kindness and listening, and work as a team to reach an agreement that will keep your family members happy and healthy for years to come.

Notes

Notes

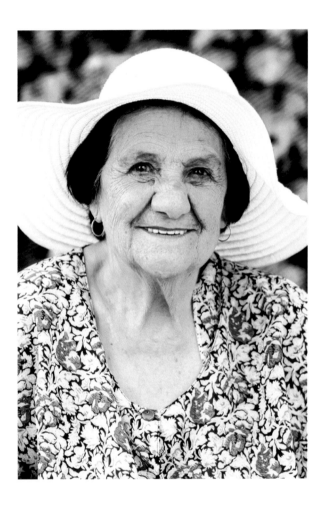

2 | *Beginning Your Search*

A s challenging as it might be to make the initial decision to move to a senior living community, more challenging decisions loom in the future for families, from discovering the kind of care required to finding the best community for you and your loved ones. Finding the right community may take some time, but the effort is well worth it.

DO THE RESEARCH

Depending on the area where you live, you may be able to choose from dozens of senior living communities (or more). This range of options can seem daunting on the surface, but if you do your homework and know what you are looking for, you can find a community that meets all of your needs.

Where to Start

A simple Google search is an excellent resource to begin

searching for the right community. Most websites will provide basic information: location, amenities, care options, and entertainment details such as activities or nearby attractions. In addition to the community's website, read online reviews to get a sense of the quality of care and staff.

Although print brochures, virtual tours, and online marketing materials all help narrow the search, nothing can beat checking out a community in person. Go on a scheduled tour with a community representative who can answer all your questions, but also pop in at other times, perhaps during a group activity or at mealtimes, so that you can see the interaction between staff and residents firsthand. Don't forget to ask one or two relatives to join the visit—you can benefit from hearing their impressions. If you are serious about a senior living community but a little unsure about a particular facility, see if you can book a temporary stay for your loved one; this can go a long way toward helping you make up your mind.

UNDERSTAND THE AVAILABLE OPTIONS IN SENIOR LIVING

If your loved one has a special medical condition, you must determine if the community can provide the support required. Some specific considerations are outlined below.

Disability, Special Needs, or Unique Medical Care

If a physical disability is present, it's important to choose a community that meets standards for both universal design and the Americans with Disabilities Act for accessibility. These are some features that indicate a community's compliance:

- Elevators
- Doorways and hallways that are wide enough to accommodate walkers and wheelchairs
- Easy-to-reach cupboards and shelves
- Bathrooms fitted with grab bars and shower chairs
- Wheelchair-accessible apartments and showers
- Emergency call systems so your loved one can call for assistance if needed
- Help for the visually impaired (find out if staff members have been trained to meet the needs of residents with low vision or complete vision loss)

"Pop in...perhaps during a group activity or at mealtimes, so that you can see the interaction between staff and residents firsthand."

Assisted Living

If your loved one needs help with any of the activities of daily living (eating, bathing, dressing, toileting, transferring/walking, and continence), it's vital to find a community that provides the right amount of personal assistance and medical care. To find out if the residence will meet the needs of your loved one, ask the following questions:

- Does the community provide medication management?
- Does a licensed nurse complete a comprehensive individualized assessment for each resident? How often are assessments reviewed?
- How many nurses are on staff? Are they on site or accessible 24 hours a day?
- Does the community have visiting physicians? Home health services? On-site therapy/rehab services?

Memory Care

Even if memory loss isn't an immediate concern, keep in mind that the incidence of dementia increases after the age 65. Below are some questions to make certain the community is equipped to deal with cognitive decline:

- Do they have a separate, secure memory care area?
- Has the staff been trained specifically to care for people with memory loss and dementia? If so, how long was the training and which skills did it cover?
- Does the community offer memory care residents special programming, such as music or art therapies and tailored recreational programs?

DETERMINE FINANCES

If finances are keeping you awake at night as you try to figure out how to pay for senior living, you are not alone. Questions about the cost and affordability of senior living are usually among the first asked by seniors and their loved ones.

First and foremost, senior living costs vary greatly across the country, which is why it's important to compare senior living costs in your local market.

These are important factors to consider when calculating the costs of senior living:

- Which services and amenities your loved one needs
- What is included in a particular senior living community's monthly rate
- How much it would cost to arrange similar in-home services

Calculating Your Current Costs

Calculating current and future living expenses is a great place to begin finding out how to pay for senior living. You can compare your loved one's current living expenses to different types of senior living, and identify any services or amenities that are not currently necessary but will be needed in the future.

Many senior living options package living expenses such as housing, meals, entertainment, utilities, transportation, and housekeeping together into a flat monthly fee. In other words, it's unnecessary to pay additional monthly expenses for services such as groceries or a vehicle registration—unless your loved one chooses to purchase those things on their own. Independent senior living does provide home health services in most communities but does not offer its own 24-hour staff.

Grab a pencil and paper or use an interactive online price calculator, like the one at www.arborcompany.com/cost-calculator, to add up the amount you pay for each of these expenses per month: mortgage or rent, utilities, home or renter's insurance, property tax, groceries, entertainment, lawn care and cleaning, maintenance or repairs, transportation and vehicle

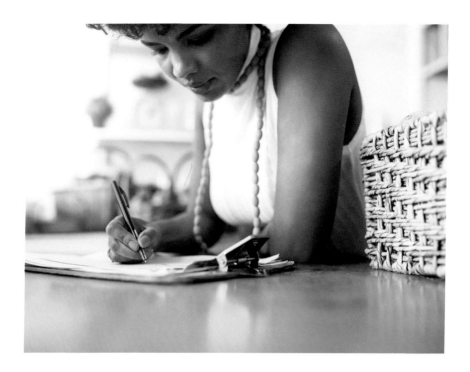

costs, home health services, and other various costs such as long-term care insurance or homeowner's association fees.

Once current living expenses are calculated down to the last dime, you can gauge the monthly amount of additional money (if any) that should be added to the budget to pay for senior living .

Calculating Costs of Independent Senior Living

Independent senior living is often the most affordable senior living option. Residents typically don't require help with everyday activities, ongoing access to medical staff, or help with medication management—so those services aren't included in monthly fees.

Independent senior living costs do include shared or private apartments, meals, laundry and housekeeping, social activities, wellness activities, and transportation services. All of the basic living expenses will be included in monthly rates. If your loved one needs home health services, such as medication management, these will not be included in the monthly rates.

Calculating Costs of Assisted Living

Assisted living is generally more expensive than independent senior living because costs include 24-hour supervision, access to medical staff, licensed on-site nurses, and medication management services.

Residents might need help with normal daily activities such as bathing, dressing, or eating. An assessment will be performed before you progress toward drafting a personalized plan to meet your loved one's particular needs. The amount of help an individual needs with activities of daily living (ADLs) will determine the best senior care option for them and, ultimately, the total monthly costs.

In addition to personal care, assisted living costs include shared or private apartments, meals, laundry and housekeeping, social programs, wellness programs, and transportation services.

Calculating Costs of Memory Care

Individuals in the mid to late stages of Alzheimer's disease and other forms of dementia often require memory care, which includes support with basic living, as well as additional support and programming for memory care.

Memory care costs include shared and private apartments, 24-hour supervision, access to licensed medical staff, skilled nurses on staff, meals, laundry, memory care programming, social activities, and transportation services. In all, memory care provides around-the-clock supervision and support to people with dementia.

Memory care costs fluctuate greatly across the country, but median monthly costs might exceed $7,000 in your area.

Calculating Costs of Skilled Nursing

Skilled nursing communities are generally for those who need more acute medical care, such as IVs, feeding tubes, ventilators, or injections, and support for all daily functions. This care is provided by a licensed nurse.

Costs include rooms, meals, housekeeping, social programs, wellness activities, and transportation services, in addition to more extensive offerings: 24-hour supervision, access to medical staff, licensed nurses on staff, and medication management support.

Overall, the median monthly cost of skilled nursing can exceed $10,000 per month.

Adding It All Up

Your first step in calculating senior living costs should be to add up current expenses, including the costs of current or future in-home senior care needs. Then, as you calculate the costs of various types of senior living—independent senior living, assisted living, memory care, or skilled nursing—you can compare those to your current costs and identify any new expenses to be incurred. Finally, remember that senior living costs vary greatly across the country, so it's important to diligently review costs in your specific region to get a true picture when calculating different types of senior living expenses.

"Observe how you are greeted by the receptionist and take note of how staff members engage with residents."

TOURING COMMUNITIES

All of your phone calls, emails, brochure reading, and online research will help you inch closer to a decision, but you won't truly get a feel for a senior living community without a tour. Here are some tips on what to look for and questions to ask during your loved one's visit to a potential new home.

Preparing for Your First Community Tour

When touring a potential community, several general things can be evaluated by simply looking around and asking the right questions. By beginning the tour with some idea of what you should be asking and looking for, you can ensure maximum comfort for your loved one at the community they may soon call home.

Staff

For most, being surrounded by staff members who are kind, sociable, and caring will trump living in a swanky environment any day. Right from the start, observe how you are greeted by the receptionist and take note of how staff members engage with residents. Do they come across as curt, cold, or dismissive? Are they friendly, nurturing, and patient? Also, be sure to ask about the staff-to-resident ratio—even the most caring workers may have little time for social interaction if they are running in all directions to meet the needs of more residents than they can handle.

Leadership

Typically, it's a good sign if the community leadership staff—managers and directors—return phone calls promptly and courteously and answer all your questions. Ask to meet the executive director and the resident care director on your tour; take note of the way they greet you and whether they reach out to residents who come across their path.

Current Residents and Families

Dropping in several times should give you a general idea of a community's social atmosphere. Are residents out and about, talking and laughing with each other, or are you left with the impression that people generally keep to themselves or sit around all day? If you feel comfortable, strike up a conversation with a resident or two for their insight on the community. Because mealtime is a great opportunity for candid conversation, you might ask to join some residents at their table for lunch or dinner. Also, ask to speak with current families who have been through the same process of placing a loved one in senior living.

Keep in mind that as people give their opinions, they are bound to talk about what they find wrong with the community. These complaints shouldn't necessarily be deal-breakers; people will naturally like some parts of their

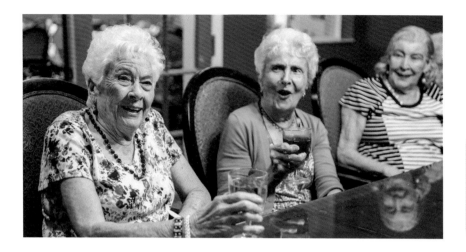

home and dislike other parts. It will be your responsibility to weigh the good versus the critical comments to form an overall impression of the community.

Amenities

In addition to housekeeping and laundry services, assisted living communities typically offer everything from wellness centers and gyms to chapels, hair salons, and concierge services. They also usually provide plenty of common spaces, such as living rooms, libraries, business and internet centers, and clubhouses.

Surroundings and Environment

There is no one standard type of senior living community; each one varies by design, ambience, and atmosphere, ranging from high-rise apartments in the middle of a bustling downtown to campus communities surrounded by trees and greenery. As you begin a tour of any community, ask yourself if the setting appeals to you and your loved one.

"Look at the community's events calendar to see if the scheduled activities appeal to your loved one."

———

If being outdoors is important, make sure there are plenty of gardens and patios, as well as places in which to sit in the sun, stroll around, or even do some gardening.

When you go inside, what is your general impression of the building itself? Do you find the decor attractive and homey, or does it have an institutional feel? Listen carefully during your visit; are noise levels tolerable? You may come across some communities that almost resemble vacation resorts; keep in mind that the fanciest places are not necessarily the best communities. Most importantly, the building should be clean, fresh smelling, and in good repair. Also, check for good natural and artificial lighting. Sunlight does wonders for the mind and body!

Although you and your loved ones should thoroughly appraise the dining hall, living rooms, and other common areas, pay particular attention to the model apartment you are shown. This brief checklist will help you evaluate the space for comfortable living:

- Can you imagine your furniture in it?
- Do suites come with a kitchenette or at least a microwave and a mini-fridge?
- Do you like the decor?

Activities and Entertainment

No senior living community will make its residents participate in an activity if they don't want to, but recognize that getting involved is often the quickest way to feel at home. With that in mind, look at the community's events calendar to see if the scheduled activities appeal to your loved one. It's usually a good sign if the community offers a diverse range of activities, including ones geared to small-interest groups—think bird watching, book clubs, or knitting clubs—as well as larger, more inclusive events, such as garden parties or holiday celebrations. Also, find out if there are scheduled outings for trips to museums and so on.

On the tour, you may be able to speak to the activity director in order to find out if the preferences of residents are considered when developing the calendar. The best communities interview new residents and families to learn about what they like to do, as well as what they used to enjoy doing. These interviews are used to build community activity calendars so everyone can find some activities of interest.

Questions to Ask Staff and Administration

Understandably, you and your loved ones will have many questions during your tour—don't be afraid to ask each and every one. After all, the answers you receive will go a long way toward making your decision. Keep some of these topics in mind as you learn more about the senior living community you are touring.

Food and Nutrition

Large senior living communities typically hire chefs and dietitians to ensure that meals are delicious as well as nutritious. If possible, find out firsthand the quality of the food by sampling a meal. Look at a monthly or weekly menu in order to see which meal options are typically offered. Determine if residents ever help with menu planning and if there are any à la carte options. If your loved one has a special diet, make sure that the kitchen can accommodate such requests.

Below are a few more questions to ask:

- When are mealtimes scheduled? Is there any flexibility around these times?
- What if a resident doesn't like items on the menu? Are there other options beyond something simple like chicken fingers?
- Are seats assigned in the dining room, or is it open/free seating?
- Can meals be eaten in private rooms or in other locations (for example, in a café)?
- Are snacks available?

Freedom to Decorate and Rearrange

For many people transitioning to senior living, the prerogative to decorate and personalize their own living quarters is high on their list of priorities. Before any contract is signed, make sure your loved one can bring their own belongings, if this is important to them. This shouldn't be a problem with most, if not all, assisted living communities; however, residential care facilities may have restrictions on the number of personal items allowed.

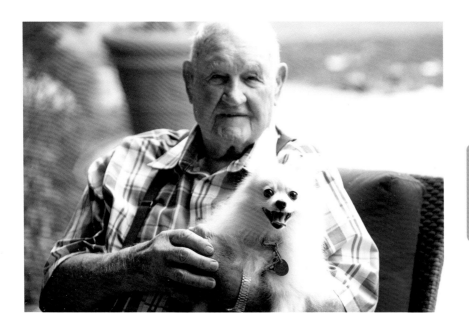

Visitation

Before you make a final decision on a particular
community, establish that friends and family can visit
whenever they like (within reason) and join their loved
one for a meal in the dining room, if desired. It's a bonus if
the community offers a separate dining room that you can
book for special occasions like birthdays. It's also a plus
if the community allows the convenience and space for a
grandchild or other visitor to spend the night in their loved
one's apartment, from time to time.

Options for Pets

If bringing the family cat or dog is a must, make a point
to inquire about pet policies. Some communities won't
allow pets at all, and some that do have restrictions on their

number or size. If a community is pet-friendly, find out if grooming and dog walking services are offered, as well as a pet coordinator who can help residents provide pet care if necessary. Take note that some "no pet" communities do have a resident dog or cat. Some may even have a pet therapy program that allows seniors to interact on a regular basis with a therapy pet (usually a dog).

Transportation

If your loved one still drives, confirm that the senior living community has a parking area for residents. If driving is no longer an option, it can make life easier and more enjoyable if the community provides scheduled transportation to doctor or hairdressing appointments as well as shopping or other activities.

On-Site Rehabilitation

For residents with recurring injuries or the aches and pains of arthritis, on-site therapeutic options such as massage, physical therapy, or occupational therapy can be convenient for rehab. Also investigate whether the community offers group exercise programs, such as tai chi, yoga, or Pilates—including seated versions for those with mobility concerns—that work to increase flexibility, balance, and strength.

Paying Attention to the Small Things

The primary features and amenities of a senior living community should be obvious during a tour. However, looking beyond the obvious—paying attention to the smaller details—is just as important for determining whether a community is right for your family. You can make a deeper assessment during a tour with these few tips:

- Request details about the specific accommodations you can expect. Ask if the unit you see on tour is similar to the one your loved one would have.
- Seek insight from friends or other family members who may think of needs you have not considered. A second opinion is invaluable to the decision about the next chapter of your loved one's life.
- Trust your instincts. Even if a place seems perfect on paper, listen to your gut if something tells you it's not right.

Narrowing Down Your List

If you tour multiple senior communities, be prepared for a degree of information overload. Understandably, you might struggle to remember what you liked and disliked about each community, or which location featured the best amenities. The Arbor Company offers a free, downloadable checklist (arborcompany.com/checklist) that can help you compare features among multiple communities in one convenient check-the-box chart. Use the checklist to organize your opinions of the toured communities to help narrow down your list.

Once you have settled on a few top choices, returning for a second tour—or simply revisiting a community at a different time of day—can give you additional information as you work toward a decision. On a second visit, pay particular mind to the attentiveness of staff, the mood of residents, the cleanliness of the communities, and other details you may have not noticed during the first tour. If you had gut feelings on your first visit, positive or negative, use the second to confirm those feelings or determine if you were mistaken.

A FINAL DECISION

Think carefully about the type of lifestyle that will truly make the senior's years more enjoyable and stress-free. For instance, if their priorities are meeting people, socializing, and entertainment, a large assisted living community in a busy metropolis might be a great fit. Alternatively, if mobility is a big concern, finding a place with on-site service providers—such as a hair salon or visiting physicians—might be top-of-mind in the overall evaluation.

Although one community may not meet all of your loved one's desires, at the very least, create a short list of must-haves versus nice-to-haves—and never look for housing based on cost alone. Sometimes a slightly higher price tag is woth the comfortable, carefree lifestyle that will allow for healthy and active senior years.

Whatever your priorities happen to be, the senior living community you choose can have a huge impact on happiness, contentment, and even health for years to come.

Notes

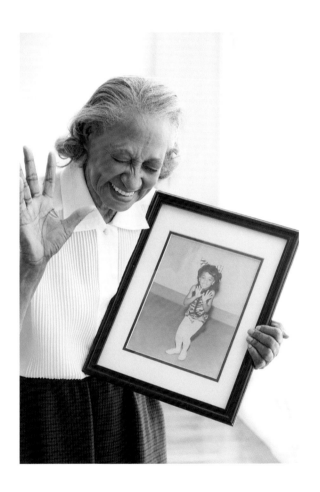

3 | *Making the Move*

After the process of deciding to move into senior living and choosing a community, the move itself might seem like the easy part of the journey. However, moving is never easy; especially for seniors, there are powerful emotions involved in leaving a home they may have lived in for decades. Take time with the move, and recognize it as a major step of the journey.

HELP YOUR LOVED ONE DOWNSIZE

The new senior living space or apartment you choose might be smaller than the size of the home where you or your loved one currently reside. If that is the case, you may need to downsize a bit. However, downsizing does not have to be something to fear. In fact, it can actually be quite liberating! Streamlining your home before packing things into boxes can feel good. (There are companies that will help with downsizing and moving, if you prefer that route.)

In order to stay organized and make the most of your downsizing, consider these tips:

- Work room by room, drawer by drawer. Resist the urge to start a new project or move onto another room before completing the one you're currently working on.
- Designate categories for every item: "keep," "donate," "give to someone special," "sell," "throw away."
- Take photos of favorite things that you won't keep; these photographs can be made into an album that you will cherish for years to come.
- If you aren't quite sure what to do with a certain item, put it aside and sleep on the decision of whether or not to keep it. Anyone can begin to make poor decisions when feeling tired or overwhelmed.
- Resist the urge to keep items in a rented storage area. You will not want to repeat this downsizing process in a few years with the items you shuffled out to your storage unit; bite the bullet and make the decisions now.
- Consider keeping holiday decorations on a reduced scale. Most senior communities encourage residents to make their apartments feel like home, and putting up a festive wreath or other items can certainly help. Just remember that you will be decorating a smaller space, so it is best to avoid toting along the seven-foot Christmas tree and opt for a small tree instead.

Although personal style and situation may dictate items that you or your aging loved one decide to bring along to the new apartment, there are a few universal categories to consider:

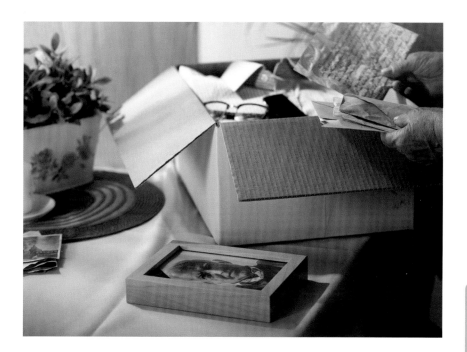

Clothing

Your loved one may be moving into a home with a smaller closet than they currently have. These are a few tips for deciding on clothing to bring:

- Take time to evaluate each piece. If it doesn't fit or hasn't been worn for a year, don't bring it.
- If your loved one is moving to a senior community in a four-season climate, don't forget to pack items for each season.
- Encourage your loved one to bring their favorite and most comfortable pieces—but consider every season.
- Don't forget to bring loungewear, pajamas, and a cozy robe.
- Go easy on shoes. It is best to bring a few pairs of comfortable shoes for daily wear, such as tennis shoes.

"Consider selling some large items and investing in smaller, more apartment-friendly furniture before the move."

- If there is a laundry service at the community, determine if you need to label clothing per any policy. Take care of this before the move so that your loved one won't have to worry about it on the first laundry day.
- If your loved one will be doing their own laundry, remember to bring a laundry basket or hamper, along with a favorite detergent and supplies.

Furniture

At most senior living apartments, residents are given an empty space ready to be filled with their own furniture. Consider a few of these ideas when loading up furniture:

- Be sure to ask about items provided by the facility and which larger pieces you may bring in.
- Measure the new apartment; keep a floor plan handy to make decisions. Nothing is more frustrating than realizing on moving day that the king-sized bed cannot fit into the new bedroom.
- Consider selling some large items and investing in smaller, more apartment-friendly furniture before the move. For example, a small loveseat and chair might suit the new living room better than a large sectional from home.

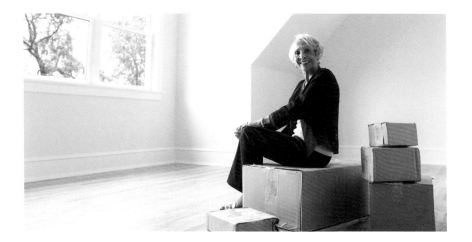

- If you have a "must come" piece, be ready for the possibility that you may have to sacrifice something else. For example, if a beloved piano is a priority, your loved one might have to forego bringing a lounge chair; there simply may not be enough space.
- Consider pieces that serve more than one function. A coffee table with drawers, for example, does double duty to enhance your storage.
- Speaking of storage, a well-placed shelving or drawer unit in the bathroom can do wonders. Drawers in the bathroom can give some extra space or eliminate the need for a linen closet.

Decor

Personal style need not diminish when moving into a senior living community! Consider these tips when packing up decor:

- Planning to hang art or photos on the walls? Keep your floor plan and measurements handy so you'll know how much you can bring on move-in day.

Making the Move

- Resist the urge to pack large pieces of art or cabinetry. In addition to furniture, these extras can make the new home seem cramped and can even become a mobility or tripping hazard.
- Speaking of tripping hazards, be wary of rugs. Unsecured rugs can cause residents to slip and trip. If you do bring rugs, make sure they are skid-proof and secured.
- Be realistic when packing up certain infrequently used items. For example, the huge Thanksgiving serving platters will only take up cabinet space in a new home.

Personal Items

Finally, encourage your loved one to bring along those extra-special items that they love, using these tips for consideration:

- Photos are great, and some should be taken along. However, there may not be room to hang all the photos that fit in the old home. Pick out favorites, and slide the others into albums that you can easily store on a bookshelf.
- Bring along your must-have items only if you know something similar is not already available. For example, consider leaving behind the coffee pot if there is a coffee service every morning right down the hall.
- Don't forget to bring a smartphone, tablet, or computer; your loved one will enjoy having one or more of these devices to stay connected. However, if you can pare down your electronics because there is a computer lab on campus, consider doing so.
- Don't forget to bring medical necessities, including medical information, prescriptions (as necessary), doctor

information, and emergency contact information. Most of these items will be collected ahead of time, but having them just in case is wise.

What Not to Pack

As you begin to finalize the packing list, remember that moving into a senior living community and a new lifestyle means letting go of certain possessions. These are a few things to consider leaving behind:

- **Cleaning supplies:** Amenities at senior living communities include regular housekeeping services. Say "so long" to deep cleaning; leave your cleaning supplies behind. Consider bringing along light supplies, such as bleach wipes or a dust cloth.
- **Oversized furniture:** Remember to keep floor-plan measurements handy as you consider which furniture to bring. Slimmed-down, apartment-friendly choices will keep the home feeling spacious and safe.
- **An entire book, puzzle, or other collection:** If your loved one has a large collection of items (books, puzzles, figurines, games, and so on), consider bringing only a few favorites. Large collections can quickly make the new space feel cramped; bringing just a few favorites can be a nod to your personality and style without sacrificing the space.
- **Extravagant jewelry:** Jewelry can certainly be an important part of your loved one's personal story and style. However, for any large collection of pricey pieces, consider putting the majority of the items in a safety deposit box or other location outside of the new apartment.

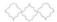

THE MOVE-IN PROCESS

After selecting a residence and putting down a deposit, your loved one will be ready to move in, but there are a few remaining steps. The move itself—arriving at the community and getting situated—requires some planning.

If your loved one has had the chance to plan ahead for the move into their new community, there will be time before move-in day to step onto their new campus to enjoy activities, meals, or other welcome opportunities. These events are the perfect way for a new resident to ease into community living by meeting key staff members and even new neighbors or friends. If possible, encourage your loved one to accept these invitations and offer to attend with them as a familiar face and touchstone of support.

For assisted living, after the initial deposit has made things official, a representative from the community will come to your home (or your loved one's home) to perform an assessment. This assessment gives the staff the opportunity to get to know the new resident a bit better and assess needs, challenges, and preferences. It is best for the community to have some of this baseline information before your loved one moves in so that the staff can be prepared to work with you from your loved one's first day at the community.

Depending on state regulations, the community may ask its new resident to visit his or her physician prior to move-in. The doctor will need to forward some state-mandated paperwork to the assisted living community. Don't worry; the assisted living community will provide you with that paperwork if it is necessary in your state.

With any type of senior living, you or your loved one will work with a representative from the community to complete some standard move-in paperwork. This paperwork typically consists of a standard rental agreement, along with other information that may ease the transition.

The move itself will be coordinated and scheduled by the team at the community. You will receive a time frame in which to arrive.

You will most likely be greeted with a welcome basket in the new apartment, and a representative from the community will give you a walk through tour of your loved one's new home. You will receive apartment keys and any wearable technology that an assisted living community may provide, such as pendants to push in case of emergency.

It's possible to put in a work request to have maintenance staff members help hang a shelf or favorite photos in the days to come. Encourage your loved one to eat amid all of the excitement; a staff representative will stop by to escort you to the dining room.

Moving day is sure to be full of excitement and stress. Families should ease their loved one's transition by simply being there to help with unpacking, coordinating movers, sitting nearby for the contract signing, or enjoying their first meal at their new home. Your familiar presence can go a long way in calming nerves and reassuring loved ones about their decision to move.

"Your familiar presence can go a long way in calming nerves and reassuring loved ones about their decision to move."

SETTLING IN

There are other ways for your loved one to make their new space feel like home upon move-in. Although every community is different, bring a bit of personality to your new space by considering a few of these tips:

- **Hang photos first:** Although putting furniture in the best spot is certainly important, hanging or displaying some favorite photos upon moving in can create a sense of welcome. Pictures will provide a reminder of home and give new neighbors and staff members something to talk about when they greet your loved ones in their apartment.

- **Enjoy a meal:** Head down to the dining room and enjoy a meal! Not only will your loved one get delicious food that they didn't have to prepare, but they will also be able to meet some new friends. It is always great to see smiling faces at dinner. If your aging loved one seems shy about eating a meal in the dining room that first day, invite yourself along. You will enjoy meeting your loved one's new neighbors, and you deserve a meal for your hard work during the move!

- **Add a welcome sign:** Something as simple as hanging a sign on the apartment door can do wonders for feeling at home. It can also be an indication that your loved one is eager to meet new neighbors.

- **Dress your windows:** Most communities will allow residents to repaint the walls in their rooms—within reason—but this may be more work than you want to undertake. An easier alternative is choosing your own window treatments. This freedom to let loved ones express themselves can add some color and style to their rooms.

- **Host friends:** Encourage your loved one to welcome friends—new and old—into his or her home as soon as possible after your move. It doesn't need to be elaborate to feel genuine; simply brew a pot of coffee (or ask for a pot to be brought in) and put some cookies on a plate. Other residents will love meeting their new neighbor, and old friends will love checking out his or her new home. Hopefully, your parent will love showing off the new space!

- **Unpack and explore:** The new space will begin to feel like home when your loved one associates it with relaxation and coziness. The best way to make a new home a safe haven is to get out and explore the new community. Encourage your loved one to take advantage of meals in the dining room as well as group activities. They will meet new friends, explore new hallways, and look forward to returning to their cozy home.

If you or your loved ones are feeling a bit disoriented after a move into the senior living community, don't worry. It is normal to feel overwhelmed about understanding assisted living for a few weeks or even months. Be honest with your family and with the staff about your feelings. You may even ask your loved one's primary care physician to drop in to see how they are adjusting.

Making the Move

Notes

Notes

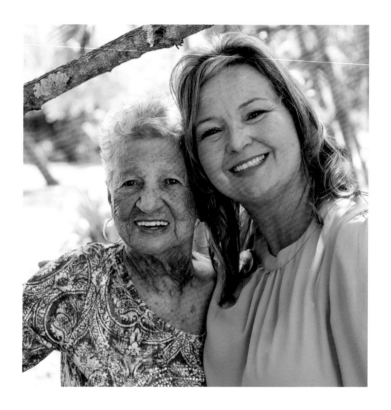

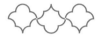

4 | *Living with Senior Living*

A move to a senior living community may be met with enthusiasm or skepticism by you or your loved ones. Undoubtedly, adjustments must be made, and one of the most difficult will be with family members who no longer fill the caregiving role they once had. Some families handle this transition well; others struggle. The best communities help residents and their families stay connected so that everyone can better adjust to senior living.

CARING AT A DISTANCE

Technology can provide a powerful impact on seniors' everyday lives. Learning how to use new technology to stay connected to family and friends brings about a host of cognitive and physical health benefits for seniors.

However, challenges may arise if seniors are hesitant to adopt newer forms of technology. Some coaxing and maneuvering may be necessary to get them to stick with it over time, but technology's ability to improve the quality of life and overall well-being of seniors will make the effort well worth your time.

A Vast Majority of Seniors Find Smartphones "Freeing"

It might be difficult to imagine Mom or Dad sending a quick text or picking up a video phone call from a great-grandchild, but helping seniors to embrace smartphone technology can result in a profound impact on their daily lives by keeping them connected to family and friends.

In fact, 82 percent of seniors who use smartphones described them as "freeing" in one nationwide study.[1] Seniors said they mostly used their phones for connection—texting, calling, and emailing. These are a few tips:

- **Be patient:** Smartphones are intuitive, but there will be a steep learning curve for seniors who have never used the technology; keep a sense of humor and try to make the learning process fun for them.
- **Reach out:** Having grandchildren, relatives, and friends text and email your parents early on will give them plenty of incentive to learn ways to use the technology to respond.
- **Go cheap:** You don't need to buy a new smartphone or tablet with an expensive data plan; an old smartphone or tablet that connects to wireless internet will allow them to call, text, email, and surf the web just the same.

---

[1] http://www.pewresearch.org/fact-tank/2015/04/29/seniors-smartphones/

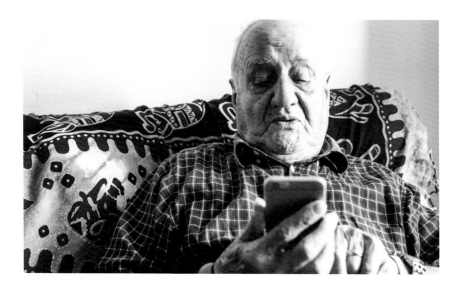

Although seniors can benefit greatly from using a smartphone or tablet, they may be reluctant to embrace new forms of technology. Stay patient and persistent until they warm up to it.

Encouraging your parents to use the available technology and resources at senior living communities is a great way to keep them connected to family and friends. Writing out instructions for how to log onto a public computer, access email, and navigate to a few websites that may be of interest might lead to more enthusiasm for technology.

Seniors on Social Media: A Growing Trend

Would you believe that social media can actually make seniors healthier and happier? A study[2] of 120 seniors in the United Kingdom found that social media training improved cognitive

---

[2] https://www.theguardian.com/media/2014/dec/12/study-finds-social-media-skype-facebook-use-beneficial-overall-health-elderly

capacity and a sense of personal competence that led to a beneficial overall impact on physical and mental health.

The power of social media is that it promotes connectedness and reduces a sense of isolation that feeds into depression and associated negative health outcomes. These are a few tips to increase the odds that seniors will embrace social media:

- **Outsource it:** Having a young family member take the reins and show your loved one how to use social media can be a great way to help them bond and learn about each other's interests.
- **Start simple:** It's important to explain to your loved ones what social media is and why people use it before helping them log on; don't expect them to know anything about social media beforehand.
- **Walk through:** Have some fun while you and your loved ones set up their Facebook profiles, and jot down notes about how to update and modify those profiles along the way. Begin building their social networks by finding and friending their family and friends.
- **Follow up:** Don't expect seniors to learn social media in one day; when you visit, continue to log onto their accounts with them, and point out new friends and messages. Soon, they'll be logging on themselves.

As with other forms of technology, seniors might be slower to adopt social media, but it has been shown to have great benefits for those who embrace it. Starting slow and being patient is a great way to keep seniors engaged. And keep in mind that it's supposed to be *fun*.

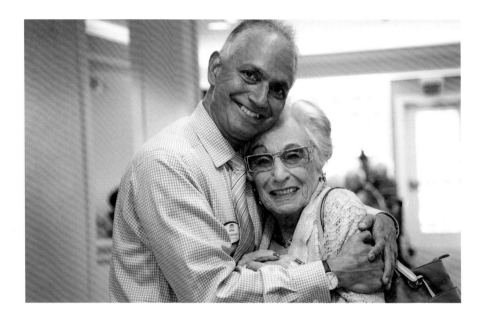

Partnering with Senior Living Staff and Administration

Family members with loved ones in senior living place a high level of trust in the administrators, staff members, caregivers, and support employees to provide the highest level of service and compassion. You and the staff at the community should be partners in doing what is best for your loved one. During the move-in process and every time you visit, take a little time to introduce yourself and say hello to caregivers and other employees. Developing rapport not only gives those employees more information about your loved one, but also encourages them to communicate with you when there is a problem—or even when there is good news.

The executive director or resident care director should be readily available to answer any questions you have regarding care, community conditions, costs, and any other concerns that arise. Don't be afraid to ask those questions—your family

"Keep in mind that everyone is striving for the same goal: the health and happiness of your loved one."

―――――

and loved one are the "customers" in this relationship, and as such, should expect the finest service possible in return for your business.

Even with the best senior living communities, disagreements may arise on occasion between residents, families, and staff. As you work to resolve any disagreements, keep in mind that everyone is striving for the same goal: the health and happiness of your loved one. Staying calm is the best way to work through problems, particularly because residents—especially those with memory problems—may already be agitated by the situation. With good communication and patience, all parties can work toward a solution that benefits your loved one.

Finally, take the time to acknowledge your loved one's caregivers, whether they are directly providing care, cooking meals, or even offering simple maintenance and housekeeping. A simple "thank you" will tell staffers their jobs are important and they are appreciated.

Notes

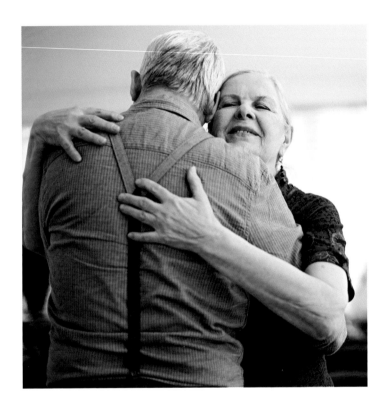

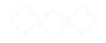

5 | *Next Steps*

The journey to senior living takes time, research, and plenty of patience. There may be tears and triumphs along the way, and hopefully, the end result will be a community where you or your loved one finds happiness, friendship, and health.

The Arbor Company brings three decades of excellence and experience to independent living, assisted living, and memory care. With more than three dozen communities in 10 states, we set the standard in senior living and are committed to our residents and their families. Take a tour today to learn more.

Even if you don't choose an Arbor community or do not live in an area where we operate, we hope you enjoyed this comprehensive guide and that you will subscribe to our blog (blog.arborcompany.com) to learn more about senior living. We also recommend these tools and resources to help you with your journey:

Senior Living Quiz – *www.arborcompany.com/quiz*
Cost Calculator – *www.arborcompany.com/cost-calculator*
Evaluating Senior Living Checklist –
www.arborcompany.com/checklist

Step-by-Step Guide to Legal Planning for Seniors –
www.arborcompany.com/step-by-step-legal-planning-ebook

Finally, if you have any questions about our senior living communities, don't hesitate to visit our online contact page (*www.arborcompany.com/contact-us*) or call us at 404-237-4026. We look forward to hearing from you!

FREQUENTLY ASKED QUESTIONS

Even after reading through our comprehensive guide, you may still have some questions. This FAQ answers some of those questions. Again, contact us (www.arborcompany.com/contact-us) if we have not covered your question in this guide.

Assisted Living

Is assisted living different from a nursing home?

Yes. The Arbor Company's assisted living communities are residential living communities that provide supportive assistance and also coordinate care with other providers in the residents' homes. As a community of caregivers, we are committed to engaging and enriching the health and spirit of our residents. We honor individuality and develop deep connections with our residents, families, and staff.

How do you know it's time for assisted living?

Change is difficult, but it's essential that you and your loved one not wait for a crisis to dictate a move into assisted living.

"An assisted living community provides healthy meals and clinical oversight, but it also provides laughter, support, and a true sense of community."

In fact, many families are surprised that assisted living makes their loved one more independent and wish they had made the decision to move sooner. Residents are offered the exact amount of support they need, without having to rely on family or friends for various tasks.

By exploring your options now, you will have more time to make an informed decision and weigh your choices. This also ensures you choose the right community for you or your loved one, versus choosing a community solely based on availability. As you consider whether now is "the time," take into account safety and quality of life. Is your loved one unsafe living at home? Does your loved one stay inside and only eat microwave dinners? An assisted living community provides healthy meals and clinical oversight, but it also provides laughter, support, and a true sense of community. It's a place where friendships are formed and life is lived to the fullest every day. And guess what? Someone else will clean up after your party!

Is the staff well-trained? How can I tell?

To get a sense of the type of care offered at a particular community, you should schedule a tour and come with questions such as these:

- How does the assisted living community staff for the resident's care needs?
- How many registered nurses, licensed practical nurses, and personal support workers are on staff? (Look for a community that has a licensed nurse on duty or on call at all times.)
- How many staffers work at any given time, including overnight?
- What is the staff members' training in such areas as safety, emergency care, first aid, mental health, residents' rights, and medication administration?

Once you've taken a tour, drop in once or twice, perhaps during a mealtime or a scheduled activity, to observe how staffers interact with residents.

Are there roommates?

Companion living options are available at most assisted living communities. Couples are also welcome!

Is anyone not eligible for assisted living?

Assisted living is not designed for adults needing 24-hour nursing services. Each state has regulations that mandate the level of care we can provide in our assisted living and memory care communities. Contact an Arbor care counselor for a personalized assessment to see if assisted living is right for you.

How can family members check in on care?

As a family member, you can relax, knowing your loved one is being cared for 24 hours a day. If an issue arises, we will notify you and work together to resolve it. Rest assured that residents' family members can visit at any time. Often, family members take residents home for visits, errands, or any other number of reasons.

Is travel still possible?

Residents may travel as they wish, so long as it is cleared by their physician.

Memory Care

What is the purpose of a memory care community?

Memory care communities offer a staff of highly trained and experienced caregivers and clinicians, while also giving seniors with dementia a safe and purpose-designed place to live and thrive. Arbor memory care communities are specifically designed to decrease wandering and increase quality of life for residents, keeping them safe and protected. Our staff is specifically trained to care for residents with Alzheimer's disease and the related diseases of dementia, including their physical, mental, and social well-being.

Even better, memory care communities serve both seniors and their families. Social workers, nurses, caregivers, and life enrichment staff are available to give you different techniques and interventions that can help make visits and bonding time more pleasant and comforting for everyone involved. A calm and happy visit can be the best gift that you or your loved one could receive.

Next Steps

"Just as the symptoms of dementia are unique to the individual, so are the interventions that work to give each affected person a high quality of life."

———————

Does the community prevent or slow down memory loss?

Although most types of dementia have no cure, many can be slowed down by early professional care and medical intervention. This can give families more time to get affairs in order, prepare for the future, and—most importantly—enjoy being a family.

Not all cases of dementia are the same; symptoms can vary from type to type, from person to person. Most seniors living with dementia will need assistance with day-to-day activities as their disease progresses. Just as the symptoms of dementia are unique to the individual, so are the interventions that work to give each affected person a high quality of life.

The silver lining in this experience is the memory care community chosen by your family. Trained professionals can assist you and your loved one, setting you free to enjoy your family relationships without the struggles and frustrations of providing medical care. Your loved one can live with dementia and maintain as much independence as the disease allows, with the right help and guidance.

What types of activities can be found in memory care?

From card games to bingo to Jenga to board games to

charades, there is always plenty of friendly competition to keep residents sharp. Trivia and other reminiscing exercises are popular among memory care residents; they can stimulate the mind and help individuals feel good about remembering. Other activities include art classes, fitness and wellness programs, social events, and special trips and outings. Routinized daily activities provide structure and a confidence of knowing what comes next.

Although there are are no known curative treatments for the primary classes of dementia, therapies—music, art, animal, aroma, storytelling, and sensory stimulation—can improve quality of life for people with dementia by lifting spirits, mending family relationships, and even extending or improving cognitive function for a time.

Therapies such as these can improve moods, may lead to moments of insight or clarity, and can help a person function to the best of their ability. These therapies are most successful when they are approached with the goal of bringing a smile or a good feeling to a person with dementia, rather than with the expectation that they will lead to long-term improvement.

Independent Living

What is independent living?

Arbor Company full-service independent living communities offer a maintenance-free lifestyle with numerous amenities and luxury services to fit your every want and need. These communities focus on providing a comfortable, independent lifestyle, but also offer peace of mind if a health issue arises. Our residents are surprised at the amount of independence they have. For example, you will still purchase toiletries such as soap, shampoo, tissue, and toilet paper.

Will I be the youngest/oldest person in the community?

Each Arbor community is home to residents of varying ages, but one thing is for sure: Age is nothing but a number. You won't notice if you are the youngest or oldest person in the community; most likely you will be too busy to ask. Communities cater to a wide range of interests, with activities that stimulate residents physically, mentally, and socially.

How "independent" is it, really?

At an independent senior living community, you have complete freedom with your time and living space. You can participate in social and recreational events in the community—or not. You can come and go as you please. As for food, independent living communities often offer custom-designed meal packages, thus allowing residents to choose a specified number of meals per day.

Is driving an option?

Absolutely! Many residents still drive their own cars, so parking is available at most communities. For those who choose not to drive, most residences offer a private bus for local shopping and day trips.

Is it possible to travel?

There are no restrictions on travel whatsoever. In fact, travel is easier and more worry-free than ever thanks to the security of knowing that your home will be safe while you're gone.

Can I drink alcohol?

Yes! In most independent living communities, alcohol is permitted. Some faith-based communities may have an alcohol-free policy, so be sure to ask when touring community options.

Can I have overnight guests?

Yes! Your apartment is just that: yours. If you would like to entertain and invite friends and family for a visit, you are more than welcome to do so.

What's the difference between independent living and a 55+ community or senior apartments?

In an independent living community, residents live in accessible apartments and have access to a number of common areas such as game rooms, libraries, business centers, and more. These communities provide numerous social and recreational activities on- and off-site. Premium independent living areas often include:

- Delicious home-cooked meals
- Transportation
- Housekeeping and laundry
- Fitness facilities
- Beauty salons
- Concierge services

There is on-site security, a 24-hour emergency help call system, and often, a nurse on staff during weekday business hours.

Senior and 55+ community apartments are similar to independent living communities, but offer few organized social activities or care services. They do offer such amenities as fitness centers, tennis courts, pools, and golf course access, and they typically have community gates and security patrol.

What happens in the case of an illness?

Many senior living options include on-site first aid and nursing care in case of emergencies. Other communities can provide nursing staff or personal companions for a fee. However, the medical services available in an independent living community are governed by state regulations, so it's important to ask questions up front about the type of assistance the community is legally able to provide.

Is there a benefit to independent living if assistance isn't needed?

At an independent living community, time isn't wasted on keeping up with housework, which means you or your loved one can devote energy to enjoying recreational activities, learning new skills, and looking after your physical, emotional, social, and spiritual well-being.

Can the environment and setting be personalized?

Independent living communities do not come in a single blueprint. You or your loved one could live in a large high-rise apartment in a downtown neighborhood or in a smaller community with a small-town feel. Units vary in size from a studio to a full apartment; in some communities, residents live in condos, townhouses, or small cottages. Also, keep in mind that regardless of the type of unit, you can furnish and decorate it as you wish; in fact, paint colors or carpeting are often customizable, just like they would be with an apartment or home rental.

What happens when the care required doesn't allow for independent living?

In some cases, one can remain in an independent living community as long as the family or a home health care provider provides caregiving. Another option is to move to an assisted living community; many independent living and assisted living communities share the same campus, making the move easier.

Senior Living

How much does it cost?

Costs for independent living, assisted living, and memory care communities vary based on location, amenities, and services, among other factors. Arbor Company communities accommodate a range of budgets.

Does Medicare cover the cost?

Medicare does not cover the rent and care costs of independent living, and its coverage of assisted living is limited to pharmacy, rehab, and other services through Medicare Part B.

Is customization available for meal plans?

Yes. Our team works hard to customize meals to specific dietary requirements, including allergies.

Next Steps

Notes

Notes

Notes